All About
BRAIN INJURIES

By Laura Flynn R.N., B.N., M.B.A., in consultation with her nurse educator associates and physicians who assisted in contributing and editing.

ISBN No: 978 1 896616 56 8

© 2011, 2017 Mediscript Communications Inc.

The publisher, Mediscript Communications Inc., acknowledges the financial support of the Government of Canada through the Canadian Book Fund for our publishing activities.

Printed in Canada

www.mediscript.net

Book and Front Cover design by:
Brian Adamson, www.AdamsonGraphics.net

BR1002010

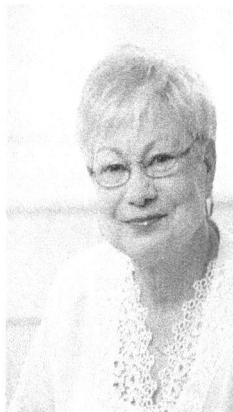

CONTENTS

INTRODUCTION

This book provides basic, non controversial and trusted information that can help a wide spectrum of readers.

The primary objective of the information is to help a person provide effective quality care to a loved one or someone in his or her care.

Your role as a caregiver could mean the older person in your care is a family member or loved one, or you may be a non family member who is helping out a friend. Alternatively, you may be a paid health worker providing quality care for a client. With this in mind, we will alternate between referring to family members, loved ones, older persons and clients.

All the information is reliable and was written by a group of eminent nurse educators who ensured the information complies with best practice guidelines and satisfies the various accreditation and regulatory bodies. Because there is so much unreliable information on the internet, you can be assured the "All About" publications are HON (Health On the Net) certified.

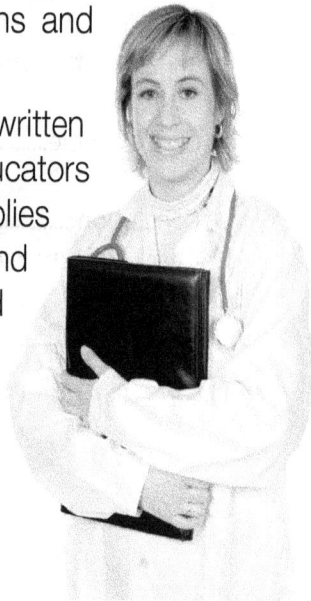

This book can be an invaluable aid to:

- A caregiver caring for a relative or friend;
- A health worker seeking a reference aid;
- A patient or person with a brain injury;
- Any person involved in health care wishing to expand his or her knowledge.

SOMETHING TO THINK ABOUT...

It takes time to succeed because
success is merely the natural
reward of taking time to
do anything well.

Joseph Ross

AN IMPORTANT MESSAGE
FROM THE PUBLISHER

Each person's treatment, advice, medical aids, physical therapy and other approaches to health care are unique and highly dependant upon the diagnosis and overall assessment by the medical team.

We emphasize therefore that the information within this book is not a substitute for the advice and treatment from a health care professional.

This book provides generic information concerning the issues around brain injuries and common sense, well-established care practices for caring for people with brain injuries.

With all this in mind, the publishers and authors disclaim any responsibility for any adverse effects resulting directly or indirectly from the suggestions contained within this book or from any misunderstanding of the content on the part of the reader.

HAVE YOU HEARD

• Mom (to her daughter after her first week at school): "What did you learn in school all week?"

Daughter: "Not much. I'm just wasting my time. I can't read, I can't write, and they won't let me talk!"

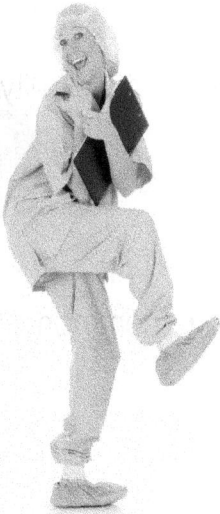

• I noticed an older woman at my neighbor's house and asked Kim, my neighbour's five-year old, if the woman was her grandmother.

"Oh, yes, she's visiting us for Thanksgiving."

"That's nice," I said. "Where does she live?"

"At the airport," Kim replied. "Whenever we want to see her, we just go out there and get her!"

Source: Unknown

HOW MUCH DO YOU KNOW?

It helps to figure out how much you know before starting. In this way you will have an idea as to the gaps in your knowledge prior to reading the content. Please circle to indicate the best answer. Remember, at this stage, you are not expected to know all the answers:

1. Brain injury always results in permanent disability.

a. True

b. False

2. Traumatic brain injuries are more common in women than in men.

a. True

b. False

3. A head injury always leads to loss of consciousness.

a. True

b. False

4. A CT scan is a:

a. Blood test

b. A test that uses a powerful magnet to show brain images

c. A special X-ray of the brain

d. A special dye used to detect tumors

5. The risk of a traumatic brain injury is highest in which groups:

a. Infants and older people

b. Teenagers, young adults, and those over 75 years of age

c. Anyone over 55 years of age

d. Teenagers and young school children

6. A person who does not respond to any type of stimulation is said to be:

a. Agitated

b. Asleep

c. Dead

d. In a coma

7. The three types of traumatic brain injury are:

a. Concussion, contusion, and skull fracture

b. Stroke, brain tumor, multiple sclerosis

c. Diabetes, cerebral palsy, and Down's Syndrome

d. Alzheimer's disease, cerebrovascular accident, cardiovascular accident

ANSWERS

1. b. True. Disability is often not permanent.

2. b. False. Statistics show that more men than women have brain injuries.

3. b. False. The majority of head injuries do not lead to unconsciousness.

4. c. Although a CT scan is a special X-ray, a dye is often used.

5. b. Statistics show that teenagers, young adults and the elderly are at highest risk.

6. d. In a coma.

7. a. Concussion, contusion and skull fracture all are types of brain injury, while the others are diseases, not injuries.

ABOUT BRAIN INJURIES

Acquired brain injury is damage to the brain due to an injury or illness that is not inherited and not something that a person is born with. Medical problems such as a stroke, disease, a brain tumor, or lack of oxygen can cause acquired brain injury.

Sometimes brain injury is the result of trauma. The cause could be a motor vehicle accident, a blow to the head during a fight, a sports accident, or a fall. This type of acquired brain injury is called traumatic brain injury, or TBI. These terms can be confusing and different organizations may use slightly different definitions for them. This review will concentrate on TBI and the care of family members or loved ones following a TBI.

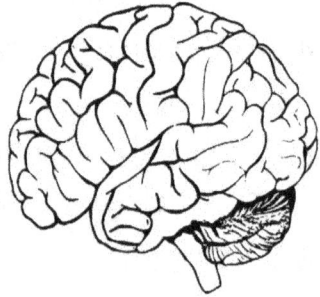

INCIDENCE

Brain injuries are very common.

- Over 50,000 Canadians sustain brain injuries each year.

- It is estimated that 5.3 million Americans live with disabilities caused by brain injury.

- Over 50,000 people die from TBI each year.

Brain injury can cause little or no permanent damage or it can leave a person with serious and permanent disabilities. Up to 40% of people with mild TBI suffer from some type of impairment that lasts for one year or longer.

RISK FACTORS AND CAUSES

Outlined below are facts about the risk factors and causes of TBI:

- TBI is about twice as common in males as in females.

- The risk of TBI is highest in teenagers, young adults, and in people who are older than 75.

- The leading cause of TBI is motor vehicle accidents.

- About half of the TBIs that occur are the result of accidents involving motor vehicles, bikes, or a person being struck by a vehicle.

- Falls are another common cause of TBIs, especially among young children and older adults. People over the age of 75 are very prone to falls. Falls are actually the leading cause of TBI in older people.

- About 20% of TBIs are caused by violent acts such as firearm usage. Assault, including child abuse, is a frequent cause of TBI in young children. Forceful shaking of infants and young children can result in TBI.

- 3% of hospital admissions from TBI are sports-related incidents.

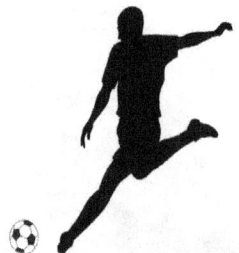

CONSIDER FOR A MOMENT ...

Have you ever known someone
with a TBI? If so, what was the
cause of the injury?
Was the cause of the injury
mentioned above?

COSTS

The cost of providing immediate and follow-up care to someone with a TBI can be very high. The cost of providing care is often long-term, as the person left with a disability may need help for the rest of his or her life. The average cost of providing care to someone with TBI over a lifetime can be well over a million dollars.

TYPES OF INJURY

The brain is the most important part of our body's control system. It controls breathing, heartbeat, and our ability to see and hear. It also controls how we move, how we think, how we feel, and how we behave. The brain is involved in everything we do and say. Brain injury can cause serious damage that may change the way we live for the rest of our lives.

There are several different types of TBI. They include the following:

Concussion

A blow to the head that makes the brain move around within the skull can cause a concussion. The person may lose consciousness for a brief time. Symptoms, such as mental confusion, poor balance, or vision problems will occur. Some concussions are more serious than others. Anyone who experiences a concussion should be seen by a doctor.

Contusion

A contusion is a more serious brain injury. In a contusion the brain is actually bruised, and the symptoms are more serious. The person who has a contusion needs follow-up medical care on a regular basis.

Skull fracture

A fracture of the skull (the bone that surrounds the brain) causes damage to the skin and bone of the skull as well as the brain. Treatment is based on the location of the fracture and how severe the fracture is. Skull fractures can cause very mild to very severe problems.

SYMPTOMS

Brain injury can cause a variety of symptoms. Outlined below are some of the symptoms that TBI survivors may experience. As each injury is unique, your family member or loved one may have any or all of the symptoms or they may have others not mentioned below:

- Memory loss that can last for just a short time or a very long time

- Trouble concentrating and thinking

- Inability to pay attention

- Poor judgment which may affect driving, work, and other aspects of everyday life

- Seizures

- Vision problems such as blurred vision, double vision, or increased sensitivity to light

- Loss of the sense of smell or taste

- Language problems

- Headaches

- Extreme fatigue

- Depression or anxiety

- Becoming angry and upset very easily

CONSIDER FOR A MOMENT ...

Have you ever known someone

with a brain injury?

If so, did you notice any of

the symptoms mentioned above?

Were there other symptoms

that are not mentioned here?

These problems may last for only a few hours. Some of them can also last for days, weeks, months, or perhaps forever. Problems with memory often last for a long time as do difficulties with attention and concentration. Even a mild injury can result in a variety of symptoms that can have a major impact on a person's life. Sometimes people do not realize that the injury has had a lasting effect on their abilities until long after the event.

MAKING A DIAGNOSIS

Some signs and symptoms of TBI may be obvious. There may be bruises, cuts, or bumps on the head and face. At other times, there may be no obvious sign of injury but the person may seem irritable, anxious, or confused. Headache, dizziness, vomiting, loss of memory, and confusion may occur. The person may become unconscious or be difficult to wake up. All persons with a head injury should be assessed by a healthcare professional.

Many older persons live alone in their own home. They may fall and injure themselves. An elderly person who suffers a TBI from a fall may act confused or display odd behaviors even if the injury is minor. When sudden symptoms of confusion or unusual behaviors appear, the older person should be assessed for a TBI.

Two tests often used to diagnose a TBI are a CT (CAT) scan and an MRI. A CT scan is a special X-ray of the brain. The person lies on a flat table that slides into a scanner, and X-rays are taken. Usually, the person receives an injection of a dye that helps to get better images of the brain. It is important to find out if he or she is allergic to the dye before it is injected.

MRI means magnetic resonance imaging. An MRI also shows images of the brain, but it is not an X-ray. The person lies very still while in a scanner because any movement might interfere with the test. There is not a lot of room in the scanner so it is important to know if the person is uneasy or frightened in small, tight places. The test is performed using a special powerful magnet so that the person should not wear anything made of metal such as metal jewelry.

Testing can be very frightening for some people. Help them to understand what is happening to them. Explain that the tests will help to find out what is wrong so that the best treatment can be given.

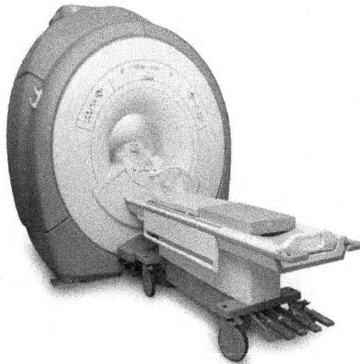

CARE CONSIDERATIONS

People recovering from TBI go through different stages or levels of recovery. Not every person will go through every stage. For example, not everyone who has a head injury becomes unconscious or goes into a coma. Recovery can take a very long time. Many people never fully recover from a brain injury.

Recovery in an elderly person may be complicated by factors such as poor stamina and the presence of various medical conditions such as heart disease, diabetes, or Alzheimer's disease. Complications are likely to be more common among the elderly.

There are different ways to assess how a person responds after a head injury. One of these ways is called the Glasgow Coma Scale. This scale assesses how well people respond with respect to opening their eyes, talking, and moving. Another way to assess someone's recovery is by using the Rancho Levels of Cognitive Functioning. This scale describes how people with TBI respond at different stages of their recovery. There is no way to know how long it will take someone to get better from a head injury or if they will ever fully recover.

The following are care issues in various stages of recovery following a TBI:

When a person is in a coma

When there is no response to stimulation the person is described as being in a coma. The unconscious person does not open his eyes. There is no response to pain or to the spoken word, even when the voice belongs to someone he knows and loves. The person may be in a coma for hours, days, weeks, or months. Or the person may never come out of the coma.

The unconscious person will not be able to meet personal needs for comfort, safety, and well-being. Proper positioning, frequent turning, skin care, and mouth care are all important aspects of care. She will not be able to eat or drink so will receive nourishment through feeding tubes and/or intravenous fluids. Intravenous (IV) means that a needle is placed in a vein in her arm or hand. The needle is attached to a clear plastic tube that is connected to bags of fluid. The fluid contains substances that are important to properly nourish the body. Since she lacks bladder control, a tube (catheter) may be placed in her bladder to collect the urine.

The person who is in a coma needs to be stimulated and encouraged to wake up. Talk to him as you provide care. Explain what you are doing and why. Nobody knows if the person in a coma can hear you or how much he or she understands. Some people who have awakened from a coma, however, have reported that they were able to hear what others said while they were in the coma. A regular schedule may be established to help stimulate the person. Try to stimulate as many senses as possible. Here are some ideas to help with this stimulation:

- Play the person's favorite music.

- Turn on the television to his favorite programs.

- Find out what type of work he did and what he enjoyed doing for fun. Talk to him about these things.

- Use touch to stimulate. This can be done by turning and positioning the person, giving him a back rub, or holding his hand.

- Allow the person to smell flowers, perfumes, or scented lotions (make sure that he is not allergic to these items).

- Bring in pictures of loved ones and place them close to his bed.

- Encourage visitors to talk to him.

Help the family to understand how important it is for them to keep talking to the person. Involve them in the person's care as much as possible. Listen to them and be supportive as they talk about their concerns.

CONSIDER FOR A MOMENT ...

Can you think of other things you

could do to help stimulate the

person who is in a coma?

When a person starts to respond

A person may come out of a coma slowly or quite suddenly. There is no way to really be sure. Observe the person carefully. The eyes may open once in a while. The first response may be from pain. As they improve, people may be able to follow simple commands such as, "open your eyes" or "squeeze my hand." Here are some things to keep in mind as your loved one starts to come out of the coma:

- She may be frightened and confused. Always talk to her and explain everything that you are doing even if you are not sure that she can hear or understand you.

- She will still need help with activities of daily living such as bathing and eating.

- Help her to understand what has happened to her. Explain any procedures that you must do. Use short, simple sentences.

- Help family and friends to deal with the person. She may respond more to certain people (maybe family and friends) than to others.

- Encourage family members to continue to stimulate her.

- Keep her safe.

When a person is agitated and confused

People may go through a stage of recovery when they become very confused and agitated (upset). Their behavior may be very strange and even hostile at times. They may have a limited attention span and may not remember their family members or friends. Even if you tell them who you are, they may soon forget. Here are some ways to help the confused and agitated family member:

- Keep the person safe. Monitor him closely. Pay attention to safety factors. Make changes before an accident happens.

- These people sometimes have a lot of energy and may need very little sleep. They can be so restless and confused that they may need a caregiver with them all the time.

- Do not take his odd behavior as a personal insult. These people are very confused and have no idea who you are or what you are doing to them.

- He may strike out at you or call you names. Try to remember that this is part of the recovery stage of head injury. He cannot help behaving this way.

- While people are in this agitated and confused stage, you must make their surroundings as quiet as you can. Speak slowly and gently. Do not shout. Do not play music or do other activities that may excite the person. Help their families and friends to understand why it is now important that they do not stimulate the person.

- Explain everything that you or others are doing to the person. These people may have a very poor memory so be prepared to explain the same thing over and over.

- Your family member will need a lot of help with activities of daily living. He may not remember what a toothbrush is or what to do with it. Be very patient and supportive.

- Help him to perform small tasks. Do not give several directions at a time. For example, do not instruct him to brush his teeth, gather towels and washcloths, and take a shower. That is too much information for him to understand. Give one instruction at a time and explain each step in the activity. For example, you could say: "Now you need to brush your teeth. Pick up your toothbrush." Once he has done so, you can say: "Put some toothpaste on your toothbrush." Remember, one step at a time. Sometimes people are too confused and agitated to do even the simplest tasks. You may need to do these tasks for them.

CONSIDER FOR A MOMENT ...

Think about your own home.

Can you identify safety risks for your family member at this stage

of recovery? What could be done to

remove those risks?

Inappropriate behaviors

At this stage, people remain confused with behaviors that are not appropriate (not exactly right for the situation). They are not agitated at this point. They may not remember how to behave when they have to go to the bathroom and may pass urine in odd places such as in a wastebasket. They have a poor memory and a poor attention span. They may not remember loved ones. They may wander away and get lost. Be aware of the following tips when caring for them:

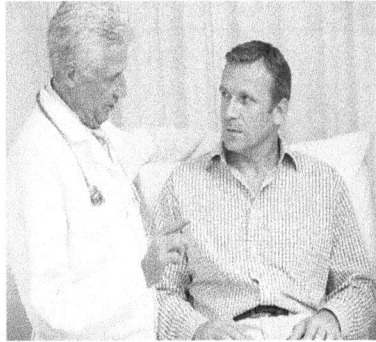

- Remind them where they are and who they are. Help them to remember loved ones. At this point, they may be able to tolerate music and other stimulation in small amounts.

- Help them to develop a regular routine. Assist them to perform activities such as bathing, eating, and dressing in the same way and at the same time each day.

- At this stage, it is best to limit the number of people that the person has to deal with. For example, it would be helpful to have consistent caregivers.

- Keep directions and tasks simple.

- Be patient and realize that you will probably need to explain the same things over and over. Be supportive!

- Although people are still confused in this stage of their recovery, different types of therapies may be started at this time. The sooner therapies can be started the better! The person may need speech therapy if she is having trouble talking. She may need physical therapy to increase her strength and to help her walk and move normally. She may need occupational therapy to learn to do her activities of daily living. She may need emotional counseling to deal with the results of head injury. She may need help finding a new job if her injuries make it impossible for her to go back to her old job.

When your loved one acts appropriately

Hopefully, your family member will recover enough to reach the stage where he is not confused or agitated and is aware of his surroundings. His behavior is nearly normal. Some disabilities may remain, however, and some of them may last forever. As the person continues to make progress, remember the following points:

- The person may be left with disabilities that are physical such as trouble speaking, walking, hearing, or seeing. These problems may be temporary or permanent.

- Some disabilities are related to thinking and emotions. The person may have ongoing memory loss. He may be more forgetful than he was before his injuries and/or may have trouble concentrating.

- Your loved one may behave differently emotionally. For example, someone who was always calm and logical may be nervous, anxious, and easily excited. They may make decisions without thinking them through.

- If people reach this stage of recovery, they behave appropriately and are able to interact with their families and friends. However, they may be depressed and irritable at times.

- At this stage, people are able to handle multiple tasks and take care of themselves.

- People with ongoing physical or emotional disabilities may have trouble keeping a job or having good relationships with family and friends. They may need emotional counseling.

- Families and friends may need help to deal with their loved ones' disabilities. The person with the injury and his family and friends must work together with the healthcare team to recover from the effects of a brain injury.

- People may not realize that they have changed after their injuries, especially if these changes are emotional. It will take a lot of work and patience to deal with these changes. It may be helpful for them to meet others who have also recovered from a head injury.

BEHAVIORIAL PROBLEMS

Problems with behavior are often the most troublesome aspects of caring for people following a brain injury. Remember, they may have many deficits that can lead to misunderstandings and frustration. They may not be able to process information well or to completely understand what is happening in any situation. There may be problems with judgment, problem solving, vision and hearing, the ability to control impulses and many other areas. They may act on impulse and may lack emotional control. They may yell, use foul language, strike out at others, and refuse to comply with treatments. These types of behaviors are disturbing to family, friends, and others providing care to the person. Sometimes it is hard to remember that the behaviors are not done on purpose.

Many different healthcare professionals can assist in developing and carrying out a plan of care for someone who displays problem behaviors as a result of a brain injury. There is, however, no easy way to change the problem behaviors. They may last a long time. In some cases they never go away. In order for the behavior to change, there must be a change in:

- The person with the brain injury,

- The people who come into contact with him or her (includes healthcare workers, family, visitors), or

- The environment.

Be flexible in your approach with your loved one. Be willing to make changes in areas that may improve her behavior. Find out what was happening before she became upset. You may be able to find a pattern and detect the cause of the outbursts. For example, does she usually lash out at others in the late afternoon? If so, perhaps fatigue is creating frustration and an inability to cope with minor stress. Try a rest period in the afternoon. Is she confused and fearful at night? Perhaps keeping a light on at night might improve the situation. Does she become startled and upset when someone approaches suddenly from behind? Remind others to approach her from the front so that she can see them.

Your loved one's plan of care may include providing feedback on inappropriate behaviors. That could involve letting him know when his behavior is not appropriate, telling him why the behavior is not proper, and explaining how his actions made you feel. Sometimes the damage from a brain injury makes it difficult for people to learn from the outcomes of their behaviors. In those cases, it is even more important to identify outside factors that may be leading to the problem behaviors and to change those where possible.

IMPACT ON THE FAMILY

TBI impacts not only the person with the injury but also the family. When a TBI occurs, family roles change. The person with TBI may have been the major wage earner in the family. If so, the resulting loss of income may create financial problems. Daily routines may change. Perhaps the injured person was the one who picked the children up after school. Now the other partner has to leave work early in order to do so.

When people are discharged from hospital and require a high level of care, they may be placed in a facility or other type of care center as they recover. Some people are discharged directly to the home. In either case, family members may be heavily involved in their care. Time demands can be enormous. These demands can have a negative effect on a person's work and personal life. It is not uncommon for family members to become depressed. They may lose contact with friends and become frustrated and angry about their situation.

The family needs to find out about and access any help that is available to them, including offers from family and friends. They need to know that it is important that they take care of themselves. They need to eat a balanced diet, keep fit, and get involved in things they enjoy. Support groups are available for survivors of brain injury as well as for their family and friends. Two good sources of information about TBIs that families can access are:

Brain Injury Association

1776 Massachusetts Ave.

NW Suite 100

Washington, D.C., 20036

(202) 296-6443

1-800- 444-6443

http://www.biausa.org

Ontario Brain Injury Association

P.O. Box 2338

St. Catharines, ON Canada L2R 7R9

1-800-263-5404

http://www.obia.on.ca

CASE EXAMPLE

John is 30 years old and recovering from a TBI. He lives at home with his wife and three school-aged children.

John is confused. Although he does not become upset like he used to, he does not always act appropriately. His memory and attention span are poor and he often forgets who his family members are.

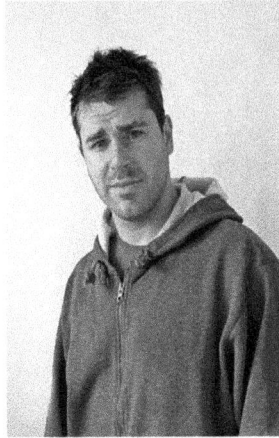

What do you think may have caused John's injury?

How could you provide the best possible care for John and his family?

YOUR ANSWERS TO CASE EXAMPLE

SUGGESTED ANSWERS TO CASE EXAMPLE

What caused John's injury?

You know that John's injury occurred as the result of a blow to the head. The injury could have been caused by a bike accident, an assault, a sports accident, or many other traumatic events. It is most likely, however, that the injury stemmed from a motor vehicle accident as motor vehicle accidents account for most TBIs.

How could you provide the best possible care for John and his family?

As John is confused and does not always act appropriately, the following guidelines may help:

- Be patient and supportive. Be prepared to repeat things over and over as needed.

- Remind him where he is, what day it is, and who his family members are.

- Establish a regular routine for bathing, rest periods, meals, and so on.

- Give him one direction at a time.

- Monitor the effect of music, the television, or visitors on his mood.

- Does he appear to enjoy these types of stimulation or do they cause him stress? Discuss your observations with the family and other healthcare team members.

- Encourage John to assist with his own care. For example, encourage him to do his personal care, to brush his teeth, and feed himself as far as he is able to do so.

- Monitor the environment for safety risks for John.

- If John appears fatigued, extra rest periods may be needed.

- Remember, each person is unique. What works in one situation for one person may not work for another.

- Follow John's care plan. If you have questions about any aspect of the care plan, discuss them with his health care professional.

- Keep family members informed and try and involve them in John's care.

- Encourage family members to take care of their own health. Listen to them as they discuss their feelings.

- Unless you've been instructed to do otherwise, be positive about John's ability to recover. The brain is an amazing structure. Sometimes even people with severe injuries make tremendous gains.

CONCLUSION

This book has mainly focused on the challenges faced by people with brain injuries, their families, and their caregivers. Remember, though, that many people do make a full recovery. Others are able to recover to the point that they can care for themselves and perhaps return to work. In working with people with brain injuries and their families, remember that "different" does not necessarily mean "worse". Sometimes people can find new strengths or build on existing ones in ways that may offset some of their challenges.

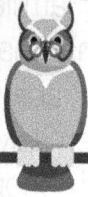

CHECK YOUR KNOWLEDGE

1. How common are brain injuries?
2. Identify three possible causes of TBI.
3. Name three types of TBI.
4. Identify the symptoms of TBI.
5. Identify several care considerations for TBI.
6. How might TBI affect the family?

TEST YOURSELF

Please circle to indicate the best answer:

1. It is best to give confused people one direction at a time.

a. True

b. False

2. The leading cause of traumatic brain injury is motor vehicle accidents.

a. True

b. False

3. The leading cause of traumatic brain injury in older people is:

a. Motor vehicle accidents

b. Assaults

c. Firearm usage

d. Falls

4. A head injury that causes bruising of the brain is called:

a. Skull fracture

b. Contusion

c. Concussion

d. Stroke

5. Which of the following statements is NOT true?

a. Over 50,000 Canadians sustain brain injuries each year

b. Over 5.3 million Americans live with disabilities caused by brain injury.

c. About 20% of traumatic brain injuries are caused by violent acts

d. About 60% of hospital admissions from traumatic brain injuries are sports-related

6. Which of the following would be most helpful in caring for a confused and agitated person recovering from a traumatic brain injury?

a. Stimulate the person as much as possible

b. Play loud music so that the person will not feel lonely

c. Advise the family not to visit until the person's condition improves

d. Talk to the person and explain what you are doing as you provide care to him or her

7. What advice would NOT be helpful to a family dealing with a traumatic brain injury?

a. Eat a balanced diet, exercise, and get involved in things they enjoy

b. Join a support group

c. Refuse offers of help from family and friends

d. Stay in contact with friends

ANSWERS

1.a. True. Give one instruction at a time and explain each step in the activity.

2.a. True. The leading cause of traumatic brain injury (TBI) is motor vehicle accidents.

3.d. People over the age of 75 are very prone to falls. Falls are the leading cause of TBI in older people.

4.b. In a contusion the brain is actually bruised, and the symptoms are more serious than in a concussion.

5.d. Only 3% of hospital admissions from TBI are sports-related incidents.

6.d. Explain everything that you or others are doing to the client. These clients may have a very poor memory so be prepared to explain the same thing over and over.

7.c. Help family and friends to deal with the client. Clients, families, and friends must work together with the healthcare team to recover from the effects of a brain injury.

REFERENCES

Bond, C. (2002). Traumatic brain injury: help for the family. RN, 65 (11), 60-67.

Brain Injury Association Network (1996). ABI facts and information. Retrieved June 11, 2003 from http://dawn.thot.net/brain/facts.htm#factsheet

Brain Injury Association of America (1999). Traumatic brain injury. Retrieved June 11, 2003 from http://www.biausa.org/Pages/types_of_brain_injury. html#symptoms

Brain Injury Association of Kentucky (2002). Brain injury. Retrieved June 7, 2003 from http://www.braincenter.org/what_brain_injury.

Falconer, J. (2000). Cognitive-behavioral brain injury rehabilitation. Quality, 7 (1), 1-4. Ontario Brain Injury Association.

Holmes, H. N. (Ed.). (2000). Handbook of diseases (2nd ed.). Springhouse, PA: Springhouse.

Lash, M. & Savage, R. (2000). Brain Injury Association of America. Questions often asked about behavior after brain injury. TBI Challenge, 4 (2). Retrieved June 10, 2003 from http://www.biausa.org/Pages/related%20articles/articles. questions%20asked%20about%20behavior.html

National Center for Injury Prevention and Control (1999). Traumatic brain injury. Retrieved June 10, 2003 from http://www.cdc.gov/ncipc/factsheets/tbi.htm

Ontario Brain Injury Association (2001). Concussion-Get the facts. Retrieved June 8, 2003 from http://www.obia.on.ca/concussion.

Pagana, K. D., & Pagana, T. J. (1999). Mosby's diagnostic and laboratory test reference (4th ed.). St. Louis: Mosby.

Page, T. J. (2001). Brain Injury Association of America. Part 4: The road to rehabilitation series. Navigating the curves: Behavior changes & brain injury. (Brochure).

Pickett, W., Ardern, C., & Brison, R. (2001). A population-based study of potential brain injuries requiring emergency care. CMAJ, 165 (3), 288-292.

Potter, P. & Perry, A. (2001). Canadian fundamentals of nursing (2nd ed.), 1577-1584. Toronto: Mosby.

Rehabilitation of persons with traumatic brain injury (1998, Oct 26-28). National Institutes of Health [NIH] Consensus Development Conference Statement. 16(1): 1-41.

Smeltzer, S. & Bare, B. (2000). Textbook of medical-surgical nursing, 1633-1673, 1675-1699). New York: Lippincott.

The Perspectives Network, Inc. (2002). Signs and symptoms of acquired brain injury. Retrieved June 8, 2003 from http://www.tbi.org/html/signs_symptoms. html

University of Missouri Health Care (2000). Concussion: Family guide to neuromedicine. Retrieved June 8, 2003 from http://www.muhealth. org/~neuromedicine/concussion.shtml